Also by T. LEE BAUMANN:

God at the Speed of Light

Window to God

The Akashic Light

The Seagull Project (fiction)

Matter to Mind to Consciousness

*Nondenominational Quantum
Spirituality Lay Manual*

The Dark Conscious (fiction)

*Sin Denominación Espiritualidad
Cuántica Manual Laico*

Medusa of Time

God at the Speed of Light: 2013 Updated
and Revised Edition

*Clearing the Air: Art of the Bowel
Movement*

The Search for Divine Justice

God Is ... (children's book)

The Drug-Free Restless Legs Syndrome Handbook

2020 Update

by T. Lee Baumann, M.D.

Baumann, T. Lee, 1950-
    The Drug-Free Restless Legs Syndrome
    Handbook
    2020 Update

Includes endnotes and index.
    ISBN: 1542527414
    ISBN-13: 978-1542527415

This book is dedicated to all sufferers of RLS.

Table of Contents

Foreword

I have suffered with a severe form of RLS for most of my adult life. The non-drug strategies employed and recommended in this handbook have been unearthed and refined out of my desperation for a reasonable night's sleep—all stemming from my varied experiences, my medical background, and the input from countless other RLS sufferers.

The approaches range from the taxing inconvenience of an isometric exercise in the middle of the night to the ridiculously simple placement of a common rubber band around the instep of your foot. Each strategy described in the pages of this text has its own merits and, conversely, weaknesses. Similarly, each individual is different. Hence, each reader will need to experiment with these various tactics to find which work best for you.

I also encourage each reader to contact me (tleebaumann@gmail.com) relative to your own drug-free successes and failures. As such, I hope to continually refine and revise this text on a regular basis to better enhance the quality of life for all RLS sufferers. Your personal feedback represents a crucial element in achieving this goal.

This revised version of my last text is the direct result of reader and patient feedback, updated research, and recent medical studies.

Here's to a good night's sleep!

Chapter 1: The Syndrome

Important note to sufferers:

For those seeking *immediate relief* of their RLS symptoms (I suspect that is most of you!), I recommend proceeding directly to **Chapter 8: Conclusions** and **Chapter 9: 2020 Update**. You may then read the preceding chapters, with their medical, historical, and supporting evidences at your leisure.

How many of us are "normal?" Just ask our significant others. Normality is a broad spectrum. Our "idiosyncracies" cover the entire spectrum. The same is true of medical disease and the gamut of medical syndromes—including Restless Legs Syndrome or RLS.

Also known as Willis-Ekbom disease (WED) or Wittmaack-Ekbom syndrome, this is a non-life-threatening malady, but one which has the capacity to make even the most pleasant personalities irritable—the direct result of many nights' "restless" or even complete lack of sleep. Although the syndrome itself is non-lethal when not associated with another disease, its effects can be. Unfortunately, our highway departments have an abundance of testimonials of affected drivers falling asleep behind the wheel. Hence, it might be wise if the medical community paid more attention to this otherwise "benign" ailment. The NIH classifies *my* RLS as severe, as I experience symptoms involving my arms, as well as my legs. As such, I believe I should share the non-drug successes that I have experienced with others. If only one or two of my treatments prove beneficial to others, then this handbook will have been worth writing.

The NIH reports the following incidence:

As many as 10 percent of the U.S. population may have RLS. …[Affecting] approximately 2-3 percent of adults (more than 5 million individuals)…the incidence is about twice as high in women. It may begin at any age…and the symptoms typically become more frequent and last longer with age.[1]

Opinions exist that drug companies exaggerate the incidence of RLS as a mechanism to further promote their drugs for its treatment.[2] Others discount this theory and suggest the figures underestimate the syndrome's prevalence. I lean toward the latter belief. I suspect a significant percentage of sufferers do not seek medical treatment, both because of its allegedly "benign" nature and the current availability of information on the Internet. Many patients will attempt simple or over-the-counter (OTC) treatments before ever considering spending money and time on a doctor's visit and/or prescription drugs. Most sufferers will self-treat by trying OTC sedatives and hypnotics, perhaps altering their smoking, alcohol, or caffeine consumption, or modifying their sleeping habits.

RLS is classified as movement disorder. It may start at any age. The syndrome is identified by the patient history. Sufferers experience uncomfortable, deep muscular sensations of the extremities, often described as "antsy," "restless," "itching," "creepy-crawling," "tingling," or the sensation of just "having to move." Along with these ill-defined sensations are often smaller muscular twitches that can escalate to more pronounced and severe jerking (the latter which can thrust the involved extremity well into the air), known as periodic limb movement of sleep (PLMS). PLMS movements may occur as often as every 15 to 40 seconds throughout the night, the latter being the most common time for their appearance.[3] Any extremity or extremities may be involved. An offending extremity one moment can transition to another extremity the next. Relief is obtained with movement, such as walking, and the symptoms return with rest. Sufferers will recognize that symptoms may occur just as commonly while seated (e.g., in an airplane) as when horizontal in bed. The National Institutes of Health (NIH) list the following criteria (all four conditions must exist) to be considered for RLS:

1. A strong urge to move your legs. This urge often, but not always, occurs with unpleasant feelings in your legs. When the disorder is severe, you also may have the urge to move your arms.
2. Symptoms that start or get worse when you're inactive. The urge to move increases when you're sitting still or lying down and resting.
3. Relief from moving. Movement, especially walking, helps relieve the unpleasant feelings.
4. Symptoms that start or get worse in the evening or at night.[4]

Symptoms

The syndrome imparts a difficult-to-describe feeling of irritability and restlessness—sometimes described as an intense itching sensation—deep within the muscles. The muscle groups can vary unpredictably from night to night, sometimes transitioning from one calf (e.g., the gastrocnemius muscle) to another—and/or involving the thighs (typically, the quadriceps)—within the course of a single night. The sensations can start, for instance, in the left calf or thigh, remain there, or spread like a plague to the right. On infrequent occasions, I have also experienced the same disturbing sensations in my upper arms (notably, the biceps).

These bizarre symptoms appear to occur most commonly at night with sleeping, during the day with napping, and annoyingly, aboard long airplane flights. The inciting mechanism is unknown.

Prevention

Other than preventing the underlying cause of a medically associated ailment (such as a neurological disease), generally no *credible, medically* researched method of *non-pharmaceutical* prevention of RLS (that I could uncover) has been established or studied. If RLS is due to any specific treatable cause (e.g., a drug or medical condition), then addressing that cause may also reduce or remove the RLS symptoms. Otherwise, current remedies focus on treating the symptoms either directly or "by targeting lifestyle changes and bodily processes capable of modifying its expression or severity."[5] Exercise in the form of walking or jogging can bring about temporary relief, but *temporary* is the key word here. Usually within minutes of returning to bed or the horizontal position, the symptoms reappear.

A good friend of mine swears to the success of a simple glass of milk before bed, but I have yet to achieve success through his exact remedy. As I will reveal in a later chapter, it appears my body requires a slightly different variation on the same theme, which feeds off of a related, albeit unknown digestive mechanism. His observation, as I will detail later, was worth investigating, and a first of many pieces to the vast RLS puzzle was set in motion.

The duration of my initial successes (nearly fifteen years, to be discussed) led me to inform various pharmaceutical representatives of *my drug-free* treatments—all to no avail. Surprise! My naivete was showing. The drug companies aren't interested in pursuing drug-free—correction—"free" treatments.

Though pharmaceutical companies promote multiple drugs for treating RLS, they are not extremely effective and are fraught with a host of potential side effects. Yet, if they might prevent undue fatigue potentially leading to an automobile accident, they should nonetheless be considered.

At the several pharmaceutical promotions I attended for RLS, drug-free therapies were *never* discussed. Again, any mention of my successes were always politely received but never seriously considered—and certainly not investigated. Hence, the reason for this handbook.

I cannot overemphasize, however, that symptoms, as well as their relief, are quite varied and individual. Still, the major treatments which I offer suggest a potential reduction of symptoms (at least for me) ranging from 50-95% for each modality alone—and close to 100% when utilized together. Of course, the success of these modalities cannot be guaranteed, nor extended to everyone.

[**Special note:** the complete proceeds from *all* my books, including this one, go to fund the multiple *God at the Speed of Light* college scholarships throughout Alabama, Mississippi, Illinois, and South Africa.]

Chapter 2: Potential Causes and Current Treatments

I must, at this point, insist that anyone wishing to attempt any treatment—those outlined in this manual or otherwise, drug or drug-free—obtain medical clearance and their physician's blessing. There are several reasons for this recommendation.

One, there are several disease states that predispose patients to RLS symptoms (see **Chapter 6**), and these treatable causes need to be addressed and/or ruled out. Successful treatment of the primary disease, if one is identified, will frequently resolve the RLS symptoms.

Disease states which are often linked with RLS include iron deficiency (prevalence as high as 34%), Parkinson's disease, kidney failure, diabetes, various types of peripheral neuropathies, varicose veins, folate deficiency, magnesium deficiency, fibromyalgia, sleep apnea, uremia, thyroid disease, attention deficit/hyperactivity disorder (ADHD), and certain autoimmune diseases including Sjögren's syndrome, celiac disease, and rheumatoid arthritis. Pregnancy has also been linked to RLS.[6] Various medications have also been implicated at causing RLS. They include some antinausea (antiemetic) drugs, antipsychotic drugs, anticonvulsants, antidepressants, sedative-hypnotic drugs, and even some common cold and allergy medications. Alcohol and tobacco have also been alleged to play a role. For the vast majority of primary RLS (i.e., not attributable to another cause), the mechanism is not known. Greater than 60% of cases suggest an autosomal dominant inheritance pattern.

Treatments

Drug therapy for RLS remains in its infancy. Various treatments exist for severe cases (e.g., where RLS prevents sleep or hinders one from performing daily activities) and include the gamut of dopamine-like drugs (e.g., pramipexole, ropinirole, rotigotine), anticonvulsants (e.g., carbamazepine), gabapentin and its precursors, the benzodiazepines (e.g., diazepam), and even opioids for severe, refractory cases. At the time of this writing, not *all* these drugs are FDA-approved for RLS. Common, drug-induced side effects from these medications may include nausea, dizziness, hallucinations, orthostatic hypotension, and daytime sleep attacks.[7]

NIH Recommendations for Prevention[8]

Excerpts from the NIH's website on RLS include the following suggestions involving prevention:

1. Some prescription and over-the-counter medicines can cause or worsen RLS symptoms.
2. Adopting good sleep habits can help you fall asleep and stay asleep...keeping the area where you sleep cool, quiet, comfortable, and as dark as possible...Going to bed and waking up at the same time every day.
3. Doing a challenging activity before bedtime, such as solving a crossword puzzle, may ease your RLS symptoms.
4. Regular, moderate physical activity also can help limit or prevent RLS symptoms.

NIH *Non-drug* Recommendations for Relieving Symptoms[9]

1. Walking or stretching
2. Taking a hot or cold bath
3. Massaging the affected limb(s)
4. Using heat or ice packs on the affected limb(s)
5. Doing mentally challenging tasks
6. Choose an aisle seat at the movies or on airplanes and trains so you can move around, if necessary.

Without wishing to sound critical, I must note from my personal experiences that I have not found these recommendations to have proved terribly helpful. Hence, I will now relate my first personal treatment success.

Chapter 3: My First Treatment Success

I must, at this point, again insist that anyone wishing to attempt this particular option get a medical clearance and their physician's blessing. Although the medical risks are minimal, some do exist. The presence of moderate to severe lower extremity arthritis (especially involving the knee), certain neuro-muscular diseases, cerebrovascular disease (e.g., history of stroke), and cardiovascular disease (e.g., history of heart attack or congestive heart failure) may prevent you from being a candidate for this next therapeutic option. This treatment involves a simple isometric exercise (though physically taxing, no repetitive movement is required). Still, healthy lower extremity joints and a healthy cerebral and cardiovascular system are required.

I further recommend that this treatment be employed only if the other, less physical treatment methods discussed later in this text fail you—and when symptoms and PLMS (periodic limb movement of sleep) are present and you cannot otherwise attain sleep without this intervention. My experience further suggests that this intervention be employed solely for *treatment*—that neither exercise nor this intervention are recommended as prophylaxis for *preventing* the symptoms of RLS. Particularly, I can attest that no exercise, including running, jogging, or stair climbing, have in any way prevented the onset of symptoms *for me*.

Since so little is known about the etiology or pathology of the disease, this isometric exercise may only serve to alleviate the symptoms until sleep occurs. My own experience indicates, however, that for the most part, the relief of symptoms lasts most of, if not all, the night. According to the NIH criteria, I suffer from the severe form of RLS since, from time to time, I endure the same signs and symptoms in my arms that I also suffer in my legs. Thus, I am confident that if these successes work for me, they may well benefit a significant number of others—and hopefully you.

Description of the isometric exercise treatment

Once the onset of symptoms has started, I have found the following protocol to be beneficial at relieving RLS symptoms:

1. Get out of bed.
2. Assume a squatting position, with the upper legs/thighs flexed at about a 30 degree angle to the lower legs/calves (see **Figure 3.1**). Use your hands to grasp a non-movable structure (dresser, table, etc.) to steady yourself as a safety mechanism to prevent falling during the exercise.
3. That's it. Maintain this isometric stance as long as possible (generally around two minutes for conditioned individuals)—and short of experiencing leg weakness due to *complete* fatigue of the leg muscles. You want to achieve the maximum safe exhaustion of the involved muscles—short of total fatigue and loss of muscular leg support. Shaking/trembling of the legs is *normal* and usually indicates that you are approaching a level of moderate fatigue. This may start almost anytime, depending on your level of conditioning. I will experience the shaking of my legs at anywhere from 60 to 90 seconds. Following the onset of shaking, I will then note a mild to moderate burning of the rapidly fatiguing muscles—again, normal. By two minutes, I am fully aware of the burning. I then attempt to maintain the position for another 15 to 30 seconds, if

possible. During these last seconds, I focus on my breathing and attempt to ignore the escalating burning. Experience will dictate the best final level of fatigue for you. When you finally attempt to resume the upright position, you may even experience that assistance with your upper extremities is helpful, depending upon the degree of leg fatigue you have achieved. [**Personal note:** When I reach the point of feeling that I cannot hold the stance any further, I count "one"...take a long inhalation followed by a prolonged exhalation...followed by "two"...again, a long inhalation followed by a prolonged exhalation...and "three"—then repeating the same three count, if at all possible. Breaking up these final breaths into allotments of three is purely a psychological ploy to divert my attention from the burning in my legs. Following these breaths, my legs can usually endure no more punishment. This is the threshold of my personal endurance and is where I stand back up—usually with great relief, but a complete absence of the RLS symptoms. This exercise protocol is usually sufficient to give me immediate and prolonged relief, usually for the remainder of the night—and it only takes about two minutes]

4. One variation that I often employ when only one leg is bothering me (not uncommon with RLS) is that I will consciously shift my position so that my weight rests slightly over the offending leg. The additional weight over the problem leg serves to shorten the duration of the exercise and targets predominately the troublesome leg.

5. **Safety first!** Despite the relative safety of this exercise regimen, perform this activity with your physician's blessing and in a safe environment free of sharp objects (e.g., nearby table corners) and preferably on a carpeted surface in the rare event that you have to sit down (or fall backwards—worst scenario) due to any inability to reassume the upright position. Although this is unlikely (it has never happened with me), I mention it solely as a precaution. [If you are unsure of your physical limitations, especially when you are first starting the exercise, have a second person at the ready to assist you, if necessary.]

6. For completeness, I will note that for the rare sufferers of RLS *of the arms*, I have obtained relief by simply doing the necessary number of pushups sufficient to

generate a burning of the muscles and to relieve symptoms. As with my experience with the legs, the relief obtained generally lasts the entire night.

7. I have found the form of above isometric exercise described for the legs to be especially beneficial for the refractory form of RLS involving the thighs (quadriceps muscles), when other treatments (yet to be described) may fail.

Do not become discouraged, particularly at first, if you find that you must repeat the exercise more than once to achieve the desired relief. Even after years of utilizing this technique, it is not unusual for me to have to repeat the treatment during the night, usually because I have not fully completed my own protocol. We're all human, and the middle of the night is not the most congenial of times to exercise—if only for 2 minutes.

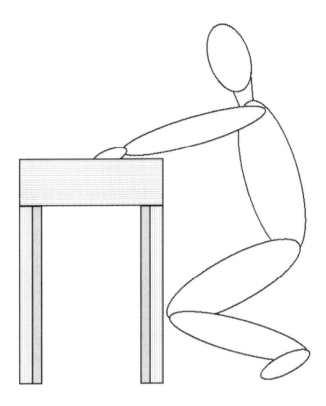

Figure 3.1 Isometric exercise stance

For travelers or theater-goers, etc., I have utilized the following alternative isometric techniques—somewhat successfully—for use in confined spaces:

1. Simply press your toes against the floor in a tip-toe stance and hold this position. This is the position of choice when it is not practical to remove your

shoes. I find that this exercise may require extended durations of time, far in excess of two minutes. The extended time requirement is the result of the inability to adequately exert the calf muscles (since you are pushing the toes against the floor, primarily by utilizing only the weight of the legs). Yet, despite the time durations required, the stance provides an appreciable relief of annoying RLS symptoms. I personally prefer the slight annoyance of maintaining this tip-toe position over that of the RLS. I cannot deny, also, that the relief typically lasts only as long as I can maintain this stance. Still, when trapped in the window seat of an airplane, I have cherished whatever relief I could obtain.

2. If you have the luxury of removing your shoes, I have obtained impressive relief, though somewhat counter-intuitive, by simply dorsi-flexing my toes (i.e., extending them toward the ceiling) and holding them in this position as pictured in **Figure 3.2**. I maintain this position as long as possible. Similar to the isometric leg technique of **Figure 3.1**, burning of the leg muscles indicates the

approach of muscular fatigue and subsequent relief of symptoms.

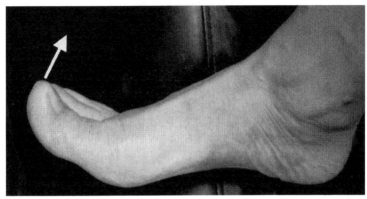

Figure 3.2 Alternative isometric technique for use in confined spaces

[**Note: If any of these techniques prove too impractical or onerous, don't be discouraged**—additional treatment and preventative approaches, which I describe in the succeeding chapters, have largely obviated the need for these unpleasant exercises.]

Chapter 4: Better than Treatment: Prevention

One day, several years ago, I noted the onset of some moderate RLS symptoms in the late afternoon. My wife and I had committed to a late dinner with my son and his wife. I would normally have not thought much about what transpired next, except that I *had* experienced significant RLS symptoms that afternoon and anticipated more that night.

Our restaurant reservation was late (for us): 8:30 p.m. When I finally climbed into bed that night (~11:30), well after my normal bedtime, I was surprised to note that I experienced no RLS sensations whatsoever that night. I made a conscious note of the tie between the absence of symptoms and the unusually late dinner.

The only thing that had changed in my daily routine *was* the late dinner. I analyzed the situation as follows:

1. A close friend swore repeatedly that drinking a glass of milk every night before bed prevented *his* RLS. His history of signs and symptoms left little doubt that he indeed did have RLS. Yet, consuming a simple glass of milk did not work for me. Yet, a physician recognizes that everybody is different.

2. The digestive process represented the obvious link between my own experience with a late dinner and my friend's benefit from his pre-bedtime milk. Further, some studies suggested a link between hypoglycemia and a worsening of RLS symptoms.[10]

3. In the medical field, the gastro-colic reflex represents a nerve reflex arc whereby food entering the stomach and the subsequent digestive process often triggers the colon to initiate a bowel movement. Similarly, the digestive process initiates the release of a host of hormones and neurotransmitters in addition to the expected digestive enzymes.

Since everyone *is* different, it is possible that an unknown digestive mechanism acted to prevent both my friend's RLS symptoms (through his glass of milk) and my own through a late supper.

4. Possible mechanisms:

    a. Gastric hormones may alleviate RLS symptoms via effects on peripheral nerves, spinal synapses (where the peripheral nerves from the body join the spinal column), or by affecting the brain's perception of RLS symptoms through some direct CNS mechanism.

b. Neuronal impulses from the stomach may somehow affect painful nerve impulses (e.g., RLS impulses) originating from the lower extremities. The stomach and small intestines receive and transmit their parasympathetic nerve signals (serving to *stimulate* GI activity) primarily from the vagus, a cranial nerve (connecting directly with the brain), whereas the sympathetic nerves (which *depress* GI activity) pass via the celiac plexus of nerves to the spinal cord (and then on to the brain). The important differentiation is that nerve impulses traversing the spinal cord (e.g., from the legs) may conceivably be attenuated by peripheral nerve impulses from other parts of the body (perhaps, in this case, the GI tract).

It is well known that certain pain sensations (traveling via pain fibers in the spinal cord) may be ameliorated by peripheral stimuli traveling via completely different and separate nerve fibers. This is the mechanism behind the *gate control theory of pain* that states that non-painful nerve impulses can close the "gates" of painful stimuli attempting to pass through to the brain (where our final perception of pain occurs). The gate control theory is theorized to be the mechanism for the pain attenuation gained by simple rubbing of a painful bruise and also transcutaneous electrical nerve stimulation (TENS). Perhaps one possible mechanism of the digestive process is that it stimulates a gate control circuit that helps to alleviate the discomfort of RLS.

[An analogy with which many readers may be familiar is that of referred pain, whereby pain in one physical area of the body affects sensation in another bodily area. A commonly recognized example is that of angina pectoris or heart pain, whereby pain originating in the heart may alter perceived sensations in the left arm—in the case of angina, actually simulating the perception of pain originating in the left arm.]

Following my initiation of the pre-bedtime meal or snack, I immediately observed a marked reduction in symptoms to a near total elimination. Over the following months, I compiled a diary which revealed a *clear* connection between a pre-bedtime meal or snack taken about one hour or so prior to bed and a marked reduction or elimination of my RLS symptoms during the night. Over time, I have become convinced that the later the meal, the less the symptoms that I experience.

The multitude of variables that influence timing of the pre-bedtime meal will undoubtedly change as time goes on—both from aging and any future medications and/or afflictions that we might later acquire. I have no doubt that you will experience a wide variation of times that work best for you. Only experimentation can dictate the optimal time of a last meal or snack. Factors that will influence the *best* timing for your pre-bedtime meal or snack will include:

1. your bedtime
2. the size of your last meal/snack
3. the time you actually *finish* your last meal/snack
4. the speed of your individual digestive process

5. any comorbid conditions
6. any medications that you are taking.

Predictably, a meal ingested immediately prior to bed will likely have a delayed onset of symptom relief (as it takes time for full digestion to begin). Similarly, a meal ingested, say several hours before bedtime, will likely have exhausted much of its RLS benefit.

In a like fashion, a larger meal may well prolong the beneficial effects of symptom relief, and a smaller meal will likely shorten the duration.

The most important recommendation I can make is to record a personal pre-bedtime meal diary of your own—at least at the beginning—and experiment. Like myself, you may be surprised at what times work best—and worst—for you.

Prevention #2:

The next observation has been attested to by other RLS sufferers, and one which I offer as a possible adjunctive practice which has repeatedly helped to alleviate—and even eradicate—my RLS symptoms.

What I have noted is a moderate to significant reduction of symptoms when my legs are exposed to cool—versus warm—air. I find that heat frequently initiates—and, if already present, exacerbates—my symptoms. During an onset of mild symptoms (antsy-itching sensations with or without mild twitching), I have discovered that placing my legs outside the bed covers, where they are exposed to the cooler ambient air, will lessen or, more frequently, completely resolve these symptoms—though not immediately. The results do impress me enough to the point where I repeatedly utilize this approach. Because of the success achieved through this simple practice, I always wear shorts to bed—never long pajama bottoms. If my body gets too cold with my legs exposed, I merely put on a comfortable light jacket, fleece, or sweater to keep my chest warm. I will sometimes adjust the thermostat to a cooler setting, if practical, to further cool the room and, hence, my legs. The exposure of my legs to this cool ambient air has a noticeable salutary effect. It generally takes at least 20-30 minutes for the exposure to cool my legs sufficiently and improve my symptoms. If the symptoms are pronounced or severe, an exercise intervention still remains as a viable next option.

For me, "cool" indicates a room temperature of no more than ~75°F—preferably less, dependent upon the degree of humidity. How cool you get your bedroom for comparable relief will vary, depending upon your own metabolic rate, your thermostat, and your bed-partner's tolerances, if applicable. The affect of the cool air on my RLS symptoms is convincing enough that I will add one further testimony supporting this method. On several occasions, I have experienced moderate RLS symptoms immediately *before* going to bed (antsy-itching sensations plus mild twitching), and I have fully anticipated having to indulge in an exercise intervention during the night. On these multiple occasions, I have intentionally placed my legs outside the bed covers immediately upon retiring—my legs fully exposed to the cooler ambient air. More common than not, the strategy works. Yet, since instituting also the pre-bedtime meal/snacks, the combined effectiveness of this simple cooling technique on the relief of *my* symptoms is substantial. It is a ridiculously simple practice that is worth trying.

Conjecture, as to the mechanism(s) behind the temperature responses for RLS have so far eluded me. Perhaps, this is another gate control theory analogy, where a non-pain stimulus (cool air or cool legs) serves to modify or negate a "painful" stimulus (RLS). If the cool air exposure has validity, perhaps this observation helps to explain the reduced incidence of RLS affecting the upper extremities in most sufferers—because we often have our arms outside of the covers when we sleep!

Yet, my observation fits the common experience of others: temperature appears to make a difference, though it is extremely varied. Whereas cold helps *my* symptoms, heat, in stark contrast, apparently helps others—at least according to the NIH's findings and recommendations (**Chapter 2**).[11] Yet, I feel compelled to include this observation with my experiences, if only to demonstrate the wide range of safe and drug-free therapies with which I encourage all RLS sufferers to experiment.

Again, history has proven that everyone's body is different and, even then, constantly in flux. As a physician, I am well aware of this truth. Hence, I would remind my readers that my personal successes may not necessarily prove beneficial for the general RLS sufferer—and certainly not those whose RLS is secondary to another disease (and for whom the primary disease needs to be treated). Trial and error will serve as your best guide. For instance, although my body and digestive processes are likely different from yours, only you can determine the optimal time for consuming a pre-bedtime meal or snack in regard to obtaining potential RLS relief. Your experiences will vary, depending upon your speed of digestion, your bedtime, your speed at falling asleep, your particular RLS gene expression and predilection, and any comorbid conditions and/or medications you may take.

Yet, for sufferers of RLS, my experiences will hopefully aid you in achieving more nights of restful sleep. This will not occur, however, without experimentation. Many sufferers will not be able to perform the isometric leg exercise because of physical limitations, such as advanced age, cerebrovascular disease, or arthritis. Others will have to experiment with the timing and size of their pre-bedtime meal/snack. Thus, experiment with the strategies I have outlined. These recommendations have at least some documented medical basis in medical physiology. Only future medical studies will decisively decide whether my observations apply to a majority of sufferers or not—and whether my hypotheses regarding potential mechanisms (to follow) are accurate or not. Unfortunately, the inability of scientific researchers (and drug companies) to make any profit by studying potential drug-free mechanisms, and the non-lethal history of the primary syndrome—except for the consequences of sleep deprivation—will cause research dollars to remain in short supply.

Still, my RLS armamentarium is not exhausted. In the next chapter I reveal my most simple treatment and prevention technique yet.

Chapter 5: My Most Successful Treatment and Prevention Technique

One afternoon I was attempting to nap following a sleepless night—the latter *not* from RLS.

I was lying comfortably on my living room sofa when my RLS struck: antsy-itching sensations and severe leg jumping. Not being in a cool room or in the immediate mood for exercise, I pondered my options.

I considered the research I had recently garnered on the gate control theory of pain for RLS (discussed previously). If gate control existed as a serious possibility, perhaps the sensory signal from another stimulus—something simple—might suffice to ward off my RLS. I peered over at a common rubber band on a nearby table, and a thought occurred to me. Could a simple rubber band stretched over my foot do anything?

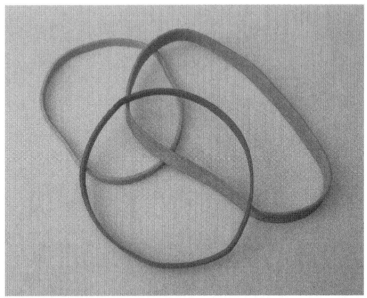

Figure 5.1 Common ¼-inch wide rubber bands

The ¼ inch wide band was just the right size for the instep of my foot. It fit comfortably about my instep—and was not at all tight (**Figure 5.2**). I laid back down and began my experiment. I observed little initial change in my symptoms and tried to ignore my RLS. It appeared that this would be a failed experiment. I remember focusing on the TV…

Then I awoke. An hour had passed. I had unexpectedly fallen asleep and napped peacefully the entire time without any further incursions from my RLS. I have subsequently repeated this simple technique on countless occasions (now extending into years) with impressive—nearly 100%—still surprising success.

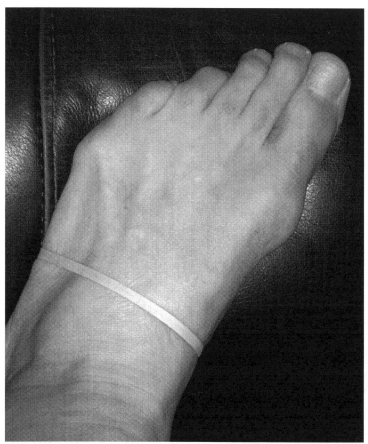

Figure 5.2 Simple rubber band around the instep of my foot

I would caution that *too tight a band* could potentially compromise the circulation to the foot—especially after several hours and for individuals for whom the circulation was already compromised, e.g., diabetics. We can all empathize with the swelling and pain that we experience after wearing new shoes that are not "broken in" or are otherwise too tight. Hence, I recommend this technique as a first choice only after a physician's evaluation and approval. Having thrown in this disclaimer, I have to say that I currently employ this simple technique as my *first choice of all my RLS treatment recommendations*. I find that, following application of the rubber band about my instep, my sensations and leg jumping continue (at a common frequency of about every 40 seconds—typical for RLS—but only for about 20-30 minutes). Hence, patience is required. After about 20 minutes, however, the intervals between my symptoms gradually lengthen, though unpredictably, until...I awake!

[**Note:** My experience dictates that the rubber band should be placed ideally about a bare foot, though a thin stocking may be tolerated.]

This experience adds impressive validity to the gate control theory of pain—i.e., the mild pressure sensation from the rubber band blocks the RLS symptoms from the leg(s), including even that leading up to violent leg jerking.

The onset of relief is so gradual with this technique that I usually find myself shifting positions during the middle of the night before realizing—once again—that the RLS symptoms had abated, allowing me to fall asleep. The technique is impressive due to its sheer simplicity and convincing success rate—and all from only the generation of a mild pressure stimulus.

Should you wish to try this technique, the pressure of the band should be moderately snug—certainly not tight and not at all uncomfortable—which might indicate impairment of the circulation. Any sign of discomfort should force you to remove the band at once and not reattempt it *with that band*. Once again, for anyone seeking to utilize this technique, procure the blessing and approval of your physician—and don't forget to take the band with you to the doctor's.

[I recommend trying first a common, ¼ inch rubber band, 3 ½ inches long, with a 7 inch total circumference, easily found in most general stores. This size band will accommodate most average-sized individuals, though stretching the band to avoid too tight a fit may be required, especially when new. I have found that I need to stretch these bands slightly for my size 11 feet. A stack of compact audio disc cases serves nicely to slightly stretch the bands, allowing me to vary the degree of stretch by the number of cases used. For instance, a stack of five cases stretching the bands over a period of a few days works perfectly for my sized feet

I also do **not** recommend wearing of the band *all the time* as a preventative measure. My experience as a physician suggests that the gate control circuit, under constant stimulation, will become tolerant of the stimulus and stop working altogether. Hence, I recommend placing of the band on your foot or feet only prior to going to bed or when the RLS symptoms occur. Having said that, my experience has also prompted me, with my level of RLS activity, to place the bands around my feet *every* night before climbing into bed—in the presence of symptoms or not. By not doing so, I inevitably find myself placing the bands on during the night and waiting the necessary 20 to 30 minutes for relief. By placing the bands on my feet before bed—even in the absence of symptoms—I obviate the waiting period.

Of special interest in support of my findings is a 2016 article from The Journal of the American Osteopathic Association. The researchers found that "targeted pressure on the abductor hallucis and flexor hallucis brevis muscles [of the foot] with an external RLS device [a simple Velcro® or hook-and-loop wrap] reduced the symptoms of moderate to severe primary RLS without the adverse effects of medication therapy."[12] Again, similar to my findings with the rubber bands, their wrap produced a striking 90% improvement in symptoms, far exceeding the results of even drug therapy (ropinirole, at 63%). If stimulated pressure over specific muscles is indeed the treatment mechanism, hence closing the RLS neuronal gate, any simple, comfortable fitting hook-and-loop wrap, strap, or rubber band will accomplish the same relative stimulation. The key to the device is comfort and pressure—whereby it won't fall off the foot.

For those for whom a proper-sized rubber band can not be found for their feet (too big, too small), a comfortable-fitting Velcro® or hook-and-loop strap fitted about the instep should offer the same benefits—soft side against the skin (**Figure 5.3**).

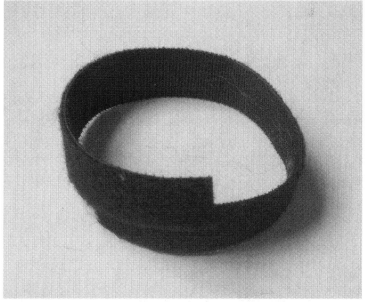

Figure 5.3 Common hook-and-loop strap

Be aware, neither a wrap, strap, nor rubber band is foolproof. A breakthrough of symptoms, even while wearing the bands, should not be cause for despair. Generally, all that is required is a repositioning of the bands, moving them as little as ¼ inch. Again, waiting the anticipated 20-30 minutes for relief is likely required for the gate mechanism to once again kick in.

Note: If choosing to use the band approach, DO NOT USE any heavy duty silicone bands (for instance, wristbands that some charities offer for donations or some entertainment venues place on your wrists for entry). These bands are too restrictive and unforgiving. Instead, experiment with just a common, 1/4-inch wide rubber band. Experiment with a variety of sizes. I have found it best if the band imparts a *moderate constrictive sensation* to the instep of the foot.

On especially bad nights, or when an obstinate breakthrough occurs, I have employed a second—and on rare occasions even a third—band, separated from the others by about a quarter inch, about the instep of the foot before achieving relief.

For sufferers of RLS, the gate control mechanism may well explain the absence of RLS symptoms with standing, walking, running, etc., where the sensory input of various other stimuli from the lower extremities block the ability of RLS-related impulses from reaching the brain. Certainly, my prolonged and repeated success of this simple rubber band technique offers substantial testimony for the gate control theory. The ability of a non-painful stimulus to close the gates on the discomfort of RLS impresses this longtime and severe RLS sufferer. I can only hope that these techniques prove as useful to you as they have for me.

[**Personal Note:** I cannot overemphasize the success I have experienced with this simple technique. Currently, I am employing this technique almost exclusively to all the other treatment options mentioned previously, with a nearly 99% success rate over the past years. Certainly, my success is not a guarantee of success for everyone, but its simplicity argues for at least trying it if you have no medical contraindications.]

Chapter 6: The Possible Mechanisms Behind RLS

The website Wikipedia.org records that approximately 2.5–15% of Americans and up to 25 percent of pregnant women suffer from RLS symptoms. In addition, RLS becomes more common and more severe with aging.[13] Yet, despite its wide prevalence, we know little to nothing of its cause. Although there are multiple drugs on the market for treating RLS, they are not very effective, and they have side effects.

In attempting to establish an etiology for the cause of RLS symptoms, researchers need to determine whether the cause is neurological (and then determine whether the nerves involved are peripheral versus central), muscular, hormonal, or even metabolic in nature.

The first hint that RLS might be linked to a direct neurological cause comes from the observation that the condition is more common in certain neurological conditions, such as Parkinson's disease, spinal cerebellar atrophy, spinal stenosis, lumbosacral radiculopathy and Charcot-Marie-Tooth disease, type 2. [14] Another suggestion for a neurological origin is the recognition that some medications for the treatment of nausea, psychosis, and depression may also worsen RLS symptoms. [15] Less clear is the observation that some chronic metabolic disease states may have associated symptoms resembling RLS. These include the forementioned states of iron deficiency, kidney failure, and diabetes to name only a few. As might be expected, successful treatment of any of the linked medical disorders may well alleviate the associated RLS symptoms. As a result, researchers surmise that any of the suspect *neurotransmitters* involved in any of the above ailments may also be involved in RLS. These suspect neurotransmitters include:

1. Amino acids such as glutamate, aspartate, D-serine, γ-aminobutyric acid (GABA), and glycine.
2. Monoamines including dopamine (DA), norepinephrine (noradrenaline, NE, NA), epinephrine (adrenaline), histamine, and serotonin (SER or 5-HT).
3. Trace amines such as phenethylamine, N-methylphenethylamine, tyramine, 3-

iodothyronamine, octopamine, and tryptamine.
4. Peptides including somatostatin, substance P, cocaine and amphetamine regulated transcript, and the opioid peptides
5. Gas signaling molecules such as nitric oxide (NO), carbon monoxide (CO), and hydrogen sulfide (H2S)
6. Other agents such as acetylcholine (ACh), adenosine, and anandamide.[16]

Wikipedia offers an excellent review of the body's *most studied* neurotransmitters:

Glutamate is used at the great majority of fast excitatory synapses in the brain and spinal cord...GABA [γ-aminobutyric acid] is used at the great majority of fast inhibitory synapses in virtually every part of the brain. Many sedative/tranquilizing drugs act by enhancing the effects of GABA. Correspondingly, glycine is the inhibitory transmitter in the spinal cord. Acetylcholine...activates skeletal muscles in the somatic nervous system and may either excite or inhibit internal organs in the autonomic system. It is distinguished as the transmitter at the neuromuscular junction connecting motor nerves to muscles...Acetylcholine also operates in many regions of the brain…Dopamine has a number of important functions in the brain; this includes regulation of motor behavior, pleasures related to motivation and also emotional arousal…People with Parkinson's disease have been linked to low levels of dopamine and people with schizophrenia have been linked to high levels of dopamine. Serotonin is…produced by and found in the intestine (approximately 90%), and the remainder in central nervous system neurons. It functions to regulate appetite, sleep, memory and learning, temperature, mood, behaviour, muscle contraction, and function of the cardiovascular system and endocrine system. It is speculated to have a role in depression, as some depressed patients are seen to have lower concentrations of metabolites of serotonin in their cerebrospinal fluid and brain tissue. Norepinephrine [acts] on the central nervous system, based on patients sleep patterns, focus and alertness…Epinephrine…plays a role in sleep, with ones ability to stay [or] become alert, and the fight-or-flight response.[17]

Since my first, most prolonged, and striking treatment success occurred through an isometric exercise routine, I will begin my initial review of potential mechanisms behind the potential RLS mechanism relating to exercise. Any immediate benefits of exercise are likely the result of exercise's metabolic byproducts. Metabolites created in skeletal muscle during exercise are chiefly creatine, adenosine triphosphate (ATP), pyruvate, and lactic acid. The first three of these metabolites are produced during *aerobic* exercise—that is, the level of exercise whereby the circulation is able to sustain the necessary levels of oxygen required by the muscle to replenish its energy sources over prolonged periods. Lactic acid and adenosine monophosphate (AMP) are produced under anaerobic conditions—i.e., when oxygen supplied to the muscles cannot keep up with demand. Other potentially important exercise byproducts to strenuous exercise (possibly relating to RLS relief) include ammonia (from amino acid catabolism of the muscle cells) and interleukin-6 (IL-6).

My personal observation that the leg muscles begin to "burn" within the timeframe of around two minutes of maintaining the isometric stance of **Figure 3.1** has medical validation as follows:

Anaerobic exercise is an exercise intense enough to trigger lactate formation. It is used by athletes in non-endurance sports to promote strength, speed and power and by body builders to build muscle mass. Muscle energy systems conditioned under anaerobic exercise conditions develop differently compared to those under aerobic exercise, leading to greater performance with short duration and high intensity activities that last from mere seconds to short of 2 minutes.[18]

Any exertion lasting *significantly* more than the magical timeframe of two minutes requires *aerobic* metabolism—i.e., a continuous oxygen supply, since the muscles require a rather constant O_2 supply to keep up with this demand over a lengthy timeframe. I certainly observe fatigue following the isometric leg stance. Although the fatigue is intense, it is short-lived and provides almost immediate relief from the RLS. I cannot rule out that any or all of the above anaerobic metabolites (i.e., lactic acid, AMP, ammonia, or even interleukin-6) contribute to the observed relief. Although my first impulse and early research was to place most of the credit on lactic acid, the following excerpt from the recent literature suggests that this is unlikely:

Researchers once attributed fatigue to a build-up of lactic acid in muscles. However, this is no longer believed. Rather, lactate may stop muscle fatigue by keeping muscles fully responding to nerve signals. The available oxygen and energy supply, and disturbances of muscle ion homeostasis are the main factor[s] determining exercise performance, at least during brief very intense exercise... During intense muscle contraction, the ion pumps that maintain homeostasis of these ions are inactivated and this (with other ion related disruption) causes ionic disturbances. This causes cellular membrane depolarization, inexcitability, and so muscle weakness.[19]

It is tantalizing to theorize that the "inexcitability" of the muscle cells' ion pumps (a refractory period) may play some role in relieving the uncomfortable RLS-generated impulses.

Yet, though many researchers do not believe lactic acid directly affects the sensation of fatigue, it cannot be ignored that *blood* lactate may rise from 1–2 mmol/L at rest to over 20 mmol/L during intense exertion.[20]

Additional research has revealed additional byproducts known as "reactive oxygen species" produced in muscles from cellular mitochondria during intense exercise and that these products impair some skeletal muscle functions. One such species is superoxide, which in turn generates hydrogen peroxide (H_2O_2). H_2O_2 in turn has a long half-life within the cell, permitting its potential diffusion into other intracellular structures or even across the cellular membrane. H_2O_2 may then react with a multitude of other molecules and subsequently activate a "wide number of signaling pathways."[21]

Other possible effects of exercise may include any combination of other metabolic and hormonal actions *upon* and/or *by* the brain, well removed from the site of the muscles themselves or their associated nerves.

Researchers have hypothesized other potential consequences of exercise, any of which may play a role in RLS. I have listed some of these candidates below:

1. A "central governor" in the brain, theorized to maintain "a safe level of exertion."
2. A reduction in the level of CNS glutamate, resulting from an uptake by the brain of exercise-generated ammonia.
3. Other yet-to-be-elucidated effects of circulating ammonia upon the brain.[22]

As I my own experiences revealed, influences other than exercise could also modify the symptoms of RLS.

Possible influence of a pre-bedtime meal/snack

If the relationship between a pre-bedtime meal/snack and my observed reduction or even elimination of RLS symptoms is real, then we would have to infer that some products or neurological responses are generated during digestion which influence the offending muscles, their nerves, or even the brain (the latter by altering our perception of the symptoms). I perceived that my isometric exercise, when it was necessary, was more effective *after* I had begun the practice of a pre-bedtime snack. Medical research offers several possible explanations. During exercise, circulation from the gut is rerouted to the muscles. Hence, not only might the effects of a pre-bedtime meal/snack stimulate the gut to produce hormones or other products capable of diminishing RLS symptoms, but any targeted exercise (such as, of the leg muscles) might intensify these effects by directly diverting the gut blood, fortified with these agents, to the involved muscles.

J.M. Polak, M.D. offers a concise summary of neuropeptides *found in the gastrointestinal tract*. I have included excerpts below of some of the leading candidates that offer potential benefits beyond the GI tract and, hence, possible roles in alleviating RLS:

Substance P has been found extensively throughout the human body...VIP [vasoactive intestinal peptide] is found in various concentrations throughout the gastrointestinal tract and may play an important role as a vasodilatory substance...Bombesin has been found in the gut, lung, and brain, and has been shown to act extensively throughout the body...In addition, enkephalin is present in the nerve fibers of the submucosa and the endocrine cells of the antral [stomach] mucosa, where it may play a physiologic role similar to morphine. Finally, neurotensin was first isolated in the brain, but has been found in highest concentrations in the gut, particularly in the ileum...

The discovery of such brain "neuropeptides," both in typical mucosal endocrine cells and in the autonomic nervous system of the gut has further consolidated the link between the gut and the central nervous system.[23]

Another potential mechanism includes the ingestion, directly, of the amino acid tryptophan (present in many foods), which the body transforms into serotonin and, subsequently, melatonin. Melatonin is well recognized as a sleep-inducing hormone. It is found in a variety of foods, including tomatoes, cherries, bananas, pineapples, oranges, grapes, rice, corn, other cereal grains, various herbs, olive oil, wine, and beer. Another candidate is, once again, serotonin, released from the GI tract as the consequence of digestion. Although serotonin is principally identified with the central nervous system, approximately 90% of the human body's total serotonin is located in the GI tract (the enterochromaffin cells).[24]

Another potential mechanism of digestion:

Anyone who has taken a nap after lunch is aware of the effect that any meal may have on our level of alertness and wakefulness. Various factors, including a diversion of blood away from the brain and to the GI tract during the course of digestion, may provoke an urge for napping and play a role, directly or indirectly, toward the alleviation of RLS symptoms.

Other candidates:

A host of other potential hormonal candidates exist which could play either major, minor, or absolutely no roles whatsoever in alleviating the symptoms of RLS during the digestive process.

These possible candidates, mentioned only for completeness, include the following (in alphabetical order):

Bombesin (activates targeted receptors in the brain)
Cholecystokinin
    (stimulates various digestive enzymes)
Endogenous opioid peptides
    (dynorphins, endorphins, and enkephalins)
Gastric inhibitory polypeptide
    (inhibits gastric activity)
Gastrin (stimulates stomach acid)
Ghrelin (stimulates appetite)
Glucose-dependent insulinotropic polypeptide
    (GIP, stimulates insulin release)
Motilin (stimulates motility)
Neuromedin B
    (NMB, regulates various secretions, cell growth, body temperature, blood pressure and glucose levels)
Neurotensin
    (interacts with other hormones and the dopaminergic system)
Secretin (stimulates secretion of bicarbonate)
Somatostatin
    (inhibits hormonal secretion and action)
Substance P (influences pain perception)
Vasoactive intestinal peptide
    (VIP, relaxes smooth muscle)

The abundance of possible candidates involved in RLS certainly complicate the investigative process. As my experiences prove, nothing is seemingly so benign as to not affect it.

Chapter 7: Alcohol and Tobacco

Alcohol is well-recognized as a neurotoxin. Hence, this text would be incomplete without at least some description of alcohol's potential, complicating role in RLS. Alcohol acts rapidly after consumption. It is absorbed directly through the lining of the stomach before even reaching the small intestine, which possesses an even greater area for absorption. The following discussion (from Wikipedia) pertains to alcohol's many potential, complicating effects throughout the body, any one of which may serve to cause, exacerbate, or alleviate RLS. Only alcohol's short-term, acute effects will be discussed.

Cell membranes are highly permeable to alcohol, so once alcohol is in the bloodstream, it can diffuse into nearly every cell.
Alcohol can greatly affect sleep (positively and negatively). Low doses of alcohol (one 360 ml (13 imp fl oz; 12 US fl oz) beer)

appear to increase total sleep time and reduce awakening during the night. The sleep-promoting benefits of alcohol dissipate at moderate and higher doses of alcohol. Rebound effects occur once the alcohol has been largely metabolized, causing late night disruptions in sleep maintenance. Previous experience with alcohol also influences the extent to which alcohol positively or negatively affects sleep…[I]nexperienced drinkers were sedated while experienced drinkers were stimulated following alcohol consumption.[25]

A common finding is that while alcohol initially causes relaxation and contributes to falling asleep, your sleep will be disrupted throughout the night. Hence, any benefit that is gained early on is lost as the night progresses.

Smoking

Not being a smoker, I can not relate any personal experiences on how smoking affects my own RLS symptoms. Yet, tobacco is a common consumable worldwide and is included by the NIH[26] as a potential causative agent for RLS. The main short-term effect of tobacco, as it might pertain to RLS, resides in its nicotine content.

Some substantiating evidence for nicotine's potential role in RLS includes the following:

Nicotine is an alkaloid stimulant. It generates a release of glucose from the liver and epinephrine (adrenaline) from the adrenal medulla. Its direct actions on the brain include the release of acetylcholine, norepinephrine, epinephrine, arginine vasopressin, serotonin, dopamine, and beta-endorphin. The variety of products that nicotine influences helps to explain its many and often contradictory actions.

Studies suggest that when smokers wish to achieve a stimulating effect, they take short quick puffs, which produce a low level of blood nicotine. This stimulates nerve transmission. When they wish to relax, they take deep puffs, which produce a higher level of blood nicotine, which depresses the passage of nerve impulses, producing a mild sedative effect. At low doses, nicotine potently enhances the actions of norepinephrine and dopamine in the brain, causing a drug effect typical of those of psychostimulants. At higher doses, nicotine enhances the effect of serotonin and opiate activity, producing a calming, pain-killing effect. Nicotine is unique in comparison to most drugs, as its profile changes from stimulant to sedative/pain killer with increasing dosages and use.[27]

Of particular interest to RLS sufferers is the finding that nicotine may produce a condition known as akathisia, a state of agitation and restlessness associated with the need to be in constant motion—a very interesting finding for RLS sufferers if a true cause-and-effect relationship is proven.

Chapter 8: Conclusions

In summary, my recommendations for the non-drug treatment of RLS are as follows, in order of my personal preference and experience:

1. **Prevention:**
   a. The pre-bedtime meal/snack, completed about one hour prior to bed appears to be ideal, at least for this RLS sufferer. The timing is contingent upon individual variation and other complicating factors (e.g., comorbid conditions and medications).
   b. Exposure of the extremities to cool air (legs outside the covers, turning down the thermostat, and turning on a fan) is the most frequently verbalized preventive measure that I hear from sufferers. I encourage sufferers to wear

an appropriate, comfortable sweater, jacket, etc. to allow them to keep their feet exposed to the cooler, ambient room air. The simple act of placing one's legs under the covers is all that is usually required to reintroduce the onset of symptoms.

c. Consider a trial of Magnesium supplementation—see **Chapter 9**.

2. Treatment, immediate, for onset of symptoms:

a. The treatment that I most frequently employ with nearly 100% success is the simple rubber band technique (**Figure 5.1**). Insure that the rubber bands are **not at all tight about the instep of the foot and elicit no more than a moderate pressure sensation or snugness.** You will need one (and rarely more) rubber band(s) about the foot of each offending leg.

[As noted previously, for those for whom a proper-sized rubber band can not be found for their feet (too big, too small), a comfortable-fitting Velcro® or other hook-and-loop strap fitted about the instep should offer the same benefits.]

The time for this gate control mechanism to take effect is in the range of about 20-30 minutes. I frequently find myself placing the bands on my feet *before* I retire, since my symptoms often begin late in the evening. Once placed, I generally leave the bands on until the following morning.

The perfect fit is one where the bands (or straps) are comfortably snug about the instep, and, when you get up the following morning, you often forget you have them on. This simple technique has proven incredibly useful for all severities of RLS involving the legs.

I will additionally utilize this technique in conjunction with any or all other therapies to reinforce or enhance their success.

   b. The quickest treatment, however, is also the most taxing: the isometric exercise technique depicted in **Figure 3.1**. I usually reserve this therapy for when my other therapies have failed me. Relief is usually complete following full *completion* of the exercise and generally will last through the night. Exceptions do occur, and you should not become discouraged if the routine requires repeating. Practice is required to achieve the optimal level of fatigue/exhaustion to successfully eradicate the symptoms for the night's duration. This is also the preferred initial step for treating the severe and often refractory RLS of the thighs.

c. For mild symptoms (e.g., antsy-itching sensations), I will attempt simple exposure of the affected extremities to the cool ambient air (legs outside the covers and/or turning down the thermostat). This approach, like the rubber band technique, takes around 20-30 minutes to achieve its effect, if is going to work. The ideal room temperature is completely dependent upon individual variation. Typically, I rarely sleep with my legs under the covers. In addition, I always place a rubber band or bands about each foot before going to bed. Experience will dictate whether one, two, or even more bands per foot work best for you. Failure of symptom relief utilizing these measures, or just the mere desire to end the symptoms quickly, should encourage you to perform the isometric exercise technique.

d. Only experimentation will dictate what combination of measures work best for you.

A typical evening for me involves the onset of symptoms with leg jerking before I retire. My typical practice involves consuming a pre-bedtime snack about one hour or less before retiring and placing the necessary rubber bands about the feet before climbing into bed. I always place the offending legs outside the covers. I always don a sweater, sweatshirt, or light jacket to keep the rest of my body warm. Generally speaking, this simple combination allows me a full night of uninterrupted sleep. Infrequent exceptions are then dealt with by employing added rubber bands or, rarely, the isometric exercise. I have been so impressed by the success of the bands + cool air exposure, that I have had to resort to the isometric technique only on the order of once every one to two months. For a severe sufferer, this success has proven priceless.

Prognosis

RLS frequently worsens with age, so those of us whose RLS is not associated with a medical condition should not expect it to ever go away. Remissions, however, are common, inexplicable, but, unfortunately, also only temporary. These remissions seldom last for more than a few days. Appreciate them, however, for what they are: gifts.

Follow-up for future book revisions

I encourage readers to E-mail me (tleebaumann@gmail.com) with both your own successes and failures and any comments regarding your responses to the strategies discussed in this handbook. I plan on making continual revisions to this text (as new editions) for the conceivable future as long as new information, recommendations, treatments, and preventive techniques become available. With your help, we can learn together how to overcome this widespread affliction.

Chapter 9: 2020 Update

I have made some new personal observations, which may or may not apply to you, but which I have found striking enough to include in this updated edition.

1.) In early 2020, I experienced a change in my life style, which resulted in an, albeit slight, increase in my nighttime gastroesophageal reflux disease (GERD). As a result, I initiated a bedtime dose of OTC antacids, containing a combination of magnesium hydroxide (the result of Mg++ oxide combining with water) and magnesium carbonate. Neither of these compounds is well absorbed. Yet, after several days, I noticed a marked reduction in my RLS symptoms. With continued observation over a several week time period, there was no doubting that I was experiencing a marked and continued reduction in my RLS symptoms. My only deduction was that the magnesium was the cause of the reduction.

As noted in **Chapter 2** of this text, I confirmed that several different medical web sites continue to suggest a link between magnesium deficiency and RLS symptoms, one of which I have listed under the "Suggested Readings" section of this book. A second therapeutic effect of Mg++ also exists by directly relaxing muscles. I doubted, however, that the level of absorbed Mg++ in my case could have exerted a direct *therapeutic* effect—except through the correction of a mild deficiency.

Detection of Mg++ deficiency is challenging. Results within the normal range can occur though the body's total stores are low. Similarly, low results can be measured in individuals without any signs of deficiency.

Approximately, 53% of the body's total magnesium is found in your bones, but an impressive 27% is found in your muscles. Further, Mg++ is the fourth most common positive ion within our cells[28]—significant figures which may explain its link with RLS.

The recommended daily allowances of magnesium are approximately 300 mg/day for women and 400 mg/day for men, intakes which may prove challenging for those of us who don't always eat properly.

I would suggest that if an oral magnesium supplement worked for me, then magnesium deficiency may be a more common cause of RLS symptoms than previously reported. Indeed, upon communicating my finding with other individual sufferers, they confirmed that their RLS symptoms also dramatically diminished or disappeared upon taking even minimal doses of magnesium. Hence, Mg++ deficiency may exist as a significant cause of RLS.

As always, in our litigious society, I would ask that you speak to your family physician before attempting to take any form of a Mg++ supplement as a treatment for your RLS, as your doctor may wish to make other important recommendations.

Assuming that you garner your physician's blessing and have no medical contraindications, you might consider a low dose of supplemental magnesium as a trial to see if you experience the same relief of your RLS symptoms as I have. There are certainly better magnesium supplements on the market than are present in most antacids to address either deficiency or to aim for its direct therapeutic affects. Magnesium citrate is probably one of the most popular and best absorbed Mg++ supplement, but your doctor will be the best judge of which supplement might work best for you.

Since my initial finding, I have subsequently switched to the better-absorbed Mg++ citrate. It is available as both a liquid and in capsule form. The lowest dosage which treats your RLS symptoms is the preferred dosage. You will also need to follow your doctor's recommendations on *when* to take the product, as Mg++ is known to decrease absorption of some medications. I have two personal observations on Mg++ supplementation:

a.) For me, taking the lowest available capsule dosage which I could find (100mg of Mg++ citrate) gave me heartburn when taken on an empty stomach. I attribute this to the disintegration of the capsule in a small, localized area of my stomach and irritating the local gastric lining. This initial problem was easily remedied, however, by merely emptying the Mg++ powder from the capsule and diluting it in water or other liquid. This practice also allows for further individualizing (e.g., reducing) the necessary dosage of Mg++ for your particular symptom relief. I found my perfect dosage to be 50 mg (half of a 100 mg capsule) diluted in 8 oz of water following lunch and 25 mg diluted in 4 oz of water following my bedtime snack.

Mg++ oxide is another choice for Mg++ supplementation, but only about 4% is absorbed compared to 25-30% for Mg++ citrate. Also, Mg++ oxide dissolves poorly in water, whereas Mg++ citrate is highly soluble in water, probably adding to the latter's increased absorption. Obviously, you can avoid the solubility problem by simply buying the liquid Mg++ citrate from the start. In the end, liquid or capsule, the end results for your RLS are the same.

b.) Mg++ citrate is also a safe, well-recognized osmotic laxative that works by drawing water into the bowel, producing softer bowel movements. It does not have the recognized harmful side affects of a stimulant laxative (like bisacodyl, the sennosides, and cascara), which can create a chemical dependency whereupon the bowel will not function without them.

As an osmotic laxative, you will want to titrate and/or time your Mg++ supplement so that you are not plagued with any social embarrassments. Hence, I personally found that my preferred dosage lay in the 50-100 mg/day dose range for Mg++ citrate, taken as either a single or even divided doses.

If you choose to take Mg++ oxide instead of citrate, the equivalent dosage would need to be on the order of 300-750 mg/day.

You might further consider supplementing your Mg++ by merely increasing your intake of foods that are high in magnesium. These include dark green vegetables (chard, spinach, kale), various nuts and seeds (pumpkin and squash), fish (mackerel and tuna), beans and lentils, avocados, bananas, and low-fat dairy including yogurt. I suggest that you experiment with these various options (e.g., liquid or capsule) and doses—the less, the better. Should you decide on the supplemental magnesium approach, note that lesser doses or less frequent doses of the product may control your individual RLS symptoms than what is recommended by the manufacturer. As an experienced M.D., I have learned that you can never assume that any seemingly innocuous, even over-the-counter (OTC) medication is truly innocuous, as everyone is different and may react differently to *any* medication. There are a host of unexpected disease states where magnesium may exacerbate the condition, including but not limited to bleeding disorders, kidney diseases, gastrointestinal ailments, and interactions with various medicines.

2.) In the preceding chapter (**Conclusions**), I recommend keeping your lower extremities exposed and cool during sleep. In the hot Summer months, however, maintaining the bedroom at a temperature to keep the legs cool enough to moderate your RLS symptoms may prove challenging. Since I remain such an advocate of a cool environment for control of RLS symptoms, I have found a simple solution to aid in this endeavor: the simple fan. Whether you may have a standard box fan, revolving fan, floor fan, or ceiling fan, any fan that can generate a gentle breeze that targets your exposed legs will prove beneficial. I have found that your nighttime room temperature does not have to be excessive for a simple fan to achieve its goal of reducing symptoms.

A slight breeze can create impressive additional cooling through two major mechanisms: 1. simple circulation of warm air away from your body and 2. evaporation of perspiration.

The change of perspiration from liquid to gas removes heat from the body, in addition to that removed by the simple circulation of air. The process is very efficient, which explains why weather forecasters are constantly giving out wind chill factors in their winter forecasts.

I continue to sleep with my legs exposed (and a fan running), on top of the covers, at night, even with my addition of magnesium!

With the new observations listed in this chapter, I am pleased to say that this severe RLS sufferer has not had to utilize any rubber bands or other treatment techniques for many months. I do *still utilize* the preventive practices of the before-bedtime snack, and I continue to sleep with my legs exposed to the ambient room air for cooling—old proven habits that are hard to break. I am crossing my fingers that some of these recommendations may work as well for you.

For those who continue to suffer, I would again encourage you to see your family medical doctor and voice your symptoms. Within the past years, I continue to hear testimonials of RLS cases that were the result of other medical conditions, such as iron deficiency anemia, listed in **Chapter 2**.

The moral is: "Don't give up hope. Continue to search for the successful individualized solution that works for you."

Suggested Readings

healthline.com "The Link Between Magnesium and Restless Leg Syndrome" <https://www.healthline.com/health/restless-leg-syndrome/link-between-magnesium-ans-rls#magnesium-and-rls>

nhlbi.nih.gov "How Is Restless Legs Syndrome Treated?" <http://www.nhlbi.nih.gov/health/health-topics/topics/rls/treatment>

ninds.nih.gov "Restless Legs Syndrome Fact Sheet" <http://www.ninds.nih.gov/disorders/restless_legs/detail_restless_legs.htm>

nhlbi.nih.gov "What Are the Signs and Symptoms of Restless Legs Syndrome?" <http://www.nhlbi.nih.gov/health/health-topics/topics/rls/signs>

WebMD.com. "Restless Legs Syndrome" <http://www.webmd.com/brain/restless-legs-syndrome>

Wikipedia.org. "Restless legs syndrome." <https://en.wikipedia.org/wiki/Restless_legs_syndrome>

Index

Endnotes

[1] ninds.nih.gov "Restless Legs Syndrome Fact Sheet" <http://www.ninds.nih.gov/disorders/restless_leg s/detail_restless_legs.htm> (September 2010) Retrieved 8 February 2015

[2] Wikipedia.org. "Restless legs syndrome" <https://en.wikipedia.org/wiki/Restless_legs_syn drome> (12 February 2015) Retrieved 20 February 2015.

[3] ninds.nih.gov "Restless Legs Syndrome Fact Sheet" <http://www.ninds.nih.gov/disorders/restless_leg s/detail_restless_legs.htm> (September 2010) Retrieved 8 February 2015

[4] nhlbi.nih.gov "What Are the Signs and Symptoms of Restless Legs Syndrome?" <http://www.nhlbi.nih.gov/health/health-topics/topics/rls/signs> (1 November 2010) Retrieved 8 February 2015.

[5] Wikipedia.org. "Restless legs syndrome" <https://en.wikipedia.org/wiki/Restless_legs_syn drome> (12 February 2015) Retrieved 20 February 2015.

[6] Wikipedia.org. "Restless legs syndrome" <https://en.wikipedia.org/wiki/Restless_legs_syn

drome> (12 February 2015) Retrieved 20 February 2015.
[7] Wikipedia.org. "Restless legs syndrome" <https://en.wikipedia.org/wiki/Restless_legs_syn drome> (12 February 2015) Retrieved 20 February 2015.
[8] nhlbi.nih.gov "How Is Restless Legs Syndrome Treated?" <http://www.nhlbi.nih.gov/health/health-topics/topics/rls/treatment> (1 November 2010) Retrieved 8 February 2015.
[9] nhlbi.nih.gov "How Is Restless Legs Syndrome Treated?" <http://www.nhlbi.nih.gov/health/health-topics/topics/rls/treatment> (1 November 2010) Retrieved 8 February 2015.
[10] Wikipedia.org. "Restless legs syndrome" <https://en.wikipedia.org/wiki/Restless_legs_syn drome> (12 February 2015) Retrieved 20 February 2015.
[11] nhlbi.nih.gov "How Is Restless Legs Syndrome Treated?" <http://www.nhlbi.nih.gov/health/health-topics/topics/rls/treatment> (1 November 2010) Retrieved 8 February 2015.
[12] http://jaoa.org/article.aspx?articleid=2531565. "Targeted Pressure on Abductor Hallucis and Flexor Hallucis Brevis Muscles to Manage Moderate to Severe Primary Restless Legs Syndrome." The Journal of the American

Osteopathic Association, July 2016, Vol. 116, 440-450. doi:10.7556/jaoa.2016.088 (1 June2015) Retrieved 29 Nov. 2016.
[13] Wikipedia.org. "Restless legs syndrome." <https://en.wikipedia.org/wiki/Restless_legs_syn drome> (27 January 2015) Retrieved 8 February 2015.
[14] Wikipedia.org. "Restless legs syndrome." <https://en.wikipedia.org/wiki/Restless_legs_syn drome> (27 January 2015) Retrieved 8 February 2015.
[15] WebMD.com "Restless Legs Syndrome" <http://www.webmd.com/brain/restless-legs-syndrome/restless-legs-syndrome-rls?page=1> (26 March 2013) Retrieved 8 February 2015
[16] Wikipedia.org. "Neurotransmitter." <https://en.wikipedia.org/wiki/Neurotransmitter> (12 July 2015) Retrieved 13 July 2015.
[17] Wikipedia.org. "Neurotransmitter." <https://en.wikipedia.org/wiki/Neurotransmitter> (12 July 2015) Retrieved 13 July 2015.
[18] Wikipedia.org. "Anaerobic exercise" <https://en.wikipedia.org/wiki/Anaerobic_exercis e> (25 June 2015) Retrieved 13 July 2015.
[19] Wikipedia.org. "Exercise physiology" <https://en.wikipedia.org/wiki/Exercise_physiolo gy> (1 June2015) Retrieved 13 July 2015.
[20] Wikipedia.org. "Lactic acid" <https://en.wikipedia.org/wiki/Lactic_acid> (19 February 2015) Retrieved 20 February 2015.

[21] Barbieri, E. and Sestili, P. "Reactive Oxygen Species in Skeletal Muscle Signaling." Journal of Signal Transduction. Vol.2012, ID 982794. <http://dx.doi.org/10.1155/2012/982794> Retrieved 13 July 2015.

[22] Wikipedia.org. "Exercise physiology" <https://en.wikipedia.org/wiki/Exercise_physiolo gy> (1 June2015) Retrieved 13 July 2015.

[23] Polak, J.M., et. al., "Neuropeptides of the Gut: A Newly Discovered Major Control System." World J. Surgery, Vol.3: Issue 4: 393-405, 1979.

[24] Wikipedia.org. "Serotonin" <https://en.wikipedia.org/wiki/Serotonin> (30 July 2015) Retrieved 3 August 2015.

[25] Wikipedia.org. "Short-term effects of alcohol" < https://en.wikipedia.org/wiki/Short-term_effects_of_alcohol> (24 July 2015) Retrieved 9 August 2015.

[26] nhlbi.nih.gov "How Is Restless Legs Syndrome Treated?" <http://www.nhlbi.nih.gov/health/health-topics/topics/rls/treatment> (1 November 2010) Retrieved 8 February 2015.

[27] Wikipedia.org. "Nicotine" <https://en.wikipedia.org/wiki/Nicotine> (3 August 2015) Retrieved 6 August 2015.

[28] Jahnen-Dechent, W. and Ketteler, M. "Magnesium Basics" https://www.ncbi.nlm.nih.gov/pmc/articles/PMC4 455825/